Diabetes

Reverse Diabetes Naturally & Safely: The Simple & Effective Changes You Can Make In Order To Reduce Blood Sugar Levels & Cure Diabetes

Jane Aniston

Table of Contents

Introduction

According to a study conducted by the American Diabetes Association in 2012, around 9.3% of the population had diabetes. Of this number, just over a third had undiagnosed diabetes. This is a very worrying statistic because having diabetes is listed as one of the seven major risk factors for cardiovascular diseases. That is the bad news - the good news however is that Adult Onset Diabetes, or Type II Diabetes is not only completely preventable but is something that can be reversed. Type I Diabetes on the other hand is harder to eradicate, but it can be brought under control.

I lived my whole life with the pall of adult-onset diabetes hanging over me because it was prevalent on both sides of my family. I get tested every year just in case the disease has progressed, but I have now taken a more proactive approach – I watch what I eat and exercise regularly, and consequently, every single year, much to the doctor's surprise given my family history, that test comes back negative.

I am going to teach you exactly what I have learned over the years and how I've managed to avoid the onset of diabetes. If you are diabetic, the information presented here will help control your symptoms. If you are not, it will help you prevent the onset of the disease. Let's get started!

Chapter 1

Understanding Diabetes

Diabetes is largely a misunderstood disease, and many people simply think that sufferers just have to make sure that they don't eat too much sugar. However, sugar is only one of the things that can cause problems when it comes to your blood glucose levels. To understand what can and cannot affect you, let us have a look at exactly how diabetes affects your blood glucose levels.

If you have diabetes, your body is either not producing sufficient quantities of insulin or it is not able to effectively use the insulin produced. What happens when you eat something is that the carbohydrates in the food you eat are broken down into glucose – the body's preferred form of energy.

This glucose enters the blood stream and the pancreas responds by releasing insulin. In a healthy individual, the insulin will help the glucose pass into the cells where it is used for energy. In a diabetic, there is not enough insulin to complete this process and the glucose builds up in the blood stream. This excess glucose is then not used as energy and is converted to glycogen in the liver, eventually causing health complications, inflammation and obesity.

The Glycemic Index

This happens with ALL carbohydrates, not just those found in sugar and that is where the Glycemic Index comes into things. Not all carbs are created equal – the less refined the carbohydrate you eat is, and the fewer natural sugars it has in it, the less impact it has on your blood glucose levels.

The Glycemic Index is based on a scale from 1-100 and shows how long foods take to impact blood sugar in comparison to pure glucose. Pure glucose is at 100 on the scale.

You should also be aware that anything that makes a food easier to digest, such as cooking, increases the glycemic value of the food, so where possible it is best to eat foods in as natural a state as you can.

If you want to keep your blood sugar on an even keel, you need to choose foods that fall within the lower half of the scale most of the time, and to avoid those foods at the very upper end completely if at all possible.

You will find that highly refined foods such as bread, sugar and rice fall into the, "foods to avoid" list. You will also find that foods that are high in fiber, protein and/or fat have a much less severe impact on blood glucose levels – providing a slow release of energy and allowing you to avoid sugar spikes and crashes.

Your Ideal Diet

Using the principles of the Glycemic Index, you can start to choose foods that will be healthy and will also help to heal your body. A good rule of thumb is to choose one portion of protein, one portion of fat and at least one to two slow-release carbs at each meal. This could mean, for example, having a steak fried in butter and served with non-starchy vegetables such as cauliflower or Brussel sprouts, or perhaps salad instead of baked potatoes or French fries.

Now, let us say that you really want that potato. You can still have it occasionally, as long as you are smart about it. Ditch the French fries – they have very little fiber in them at all. Instead, stick to a baked potato.

Make sure that all the other vegetables on your plate are very low GI to compensate and ensure that you do have fat and protein with your potato in order to reduce the glycemic load even further.

Whilst there are foods that you should definitely avoid, you can enjoy the occasional treat as long as it won't lead to an out and out binge. For example, I do like to have cake every now and then – what I do, however, is just have a small piece and always either eat it after a healthy meal or with a glass of full-cream milk. (The fat and protein in the milk help to reduce the glycemic load of the meal overall.)

Eat Only as Much as You Need

That said, even if you are eating a completely healthy diet, if you take in more calories than you need on a daily basis, you are going to gain weight. It is important that you do watch what you eat and learn to eat only when hungry.

There are those who advocate grazing throughout the day – that is, having 6 smaller meals instead of 3 meals, in order to keep blood sugar levels even but I do think that this is a matter of personal preference. I find that if you eat the right combinations at mealtimes, three meals a day is more than enough.

If you are concerned about getting hungry between meals, keep a snack pack handy, just make sure that it is a healthy one. Trail mix, without added sugar and a plain, unsweetened yogurt are a good option. An apple and some nut butter without added sugar is another. Almonds with some berries can also make a great snack option when you need lots of energy.

Chapter 2

Symptoms of Diabetes and What to Do About Them

The main problem when it comes to diagnosing diabetes is that it may not present symptoms until the condition is quite far advanced. That is why it is essential to get screened annually if there is a strong family history of the disease, especially if you are overweight.

Symptoms to Look Out For

How well do you sleep at night?

Insomnia can be both a symptom of diabetes and a causal factor. If you usually get fewer than 5 hours of uninterrupted sleep a day, you run a higher chance of developing diabetes. Lack of sleep puts undue stress on the body and the more sleep-deprived you are, the harder it is for hormones, like Ghrelin, the hunger hormone, to work. You are more likely to choose the less healthy options and to eat more. Insomnia could also be a symptom that you have uncontrolled blood sugar levels as plunging sugar levels can interfere with your ability to sleep deeply.

Are you the mother of a baby that was big when born?

If your child weighed over 4kg at birth, you might have developed gestational diabetes when pregnant. This will generally right itself once the baby is born but can increase your risk of developing adult onset diabetes.

Do you have a high LDL cholesterol count?

If this is more than five, this could indicate that there is a problem with the way the insulin in your body is functioning. Insulin controls not only how and when glucose is burnt but also how we use our fat stores. If your LDL cholesterol levels are high, you need to start bringing them down as much as possible.

Have You Got Polycystic Ovary Syndrome? Are you a man with low testosterone levels?

In both cases, these conditions could put you at higher risk of developing adult onset diabetes.

Are you thirstier than normal? Do you need to pee more often than you used to?

Fortunately, these are signs that do appear earlier in the disease and this should be taken seriously. This is your body's attempt to try and flush out excess glucose in the blood stream.

Do you have recurrent thrush or itchy genitalia?

All women have problems with thrush every now and again but the disease really thrives in a system where the sugar levels are constantly elevated. If you keep getting thrush, it may be time to get yourself checked out.

How fast do wounds on your body heal and do you pick up every bug?

People with diabetes find that their wounds take a lot longer to heal. Your immune system is being attacked on two fronts here – high levels of glucose in the bloodstream suppress the immune system and the same can be said for insulin.

Is your vision blurry?

Believe it or not, my mother found out that she probably had diabetes when getting glasses. Her optometrist advised her to get checked out because of the deterioration in her vision.

Are you always tired, no matter how much sleep you get?

If you seem to be tired all the time without good reason, it could be a sign that you blood sugar levels are out of whack. Do yourself a favor and check it out before writing it off to stress.

Do you have an "apple" shape?

You do not have to be overweight to develop diabetes but seeing where your excess weight lies is one of the best ways to see whether or not you are at risk for diabetes. Weight that accumulates around the abdomen, especially weight that is really hard to shift, could be a symptom of insulin resistance developing.

A dramatic change in weight for seemingly no reason.

If you have recently started losing or gaining a lot of weight without trying, you should get yourself checked out.

Do your extremities often feel numb or tingly?

This could be a symptom of bad circulation but could also be a symptom nerve damage caused by diabetes. Diabetics especially need to be careful of injuring their hands and feet because they tend to be less sensitive to pain. A friend's father had uncontrolled diabetes and stepped on a nail. He didn't feel it and didn't realize it. The wound became infected and gangrene set in. He eventually had to have the foot removed.

Chapter 3

Foods to Include in Your Diet

to Beat Diabetes

As mentioned earlier, the emphasis should be on food that releases a slow, steady stream of energy rather than one big flash that fizzle out. Here is my top list of foods that help to beat diabetes:

Oatmeal

Choose whole oats that have been minimally processed for the best results. In a pinch, though, you can get quick cooking oats as long as they are unsweetened. To up the fiber content of the quick cooking oats, add in some oat bran as well. Raw oats are best so do look at making your own granola and eating it raw. Allow it to soak in milk overnight so that it is deliciously soft in the morning. Also, make a determined effort to add oats into your day to day cooking. I replace half the breadcrumbs in my meatballs with oats, add them to smoothies, and use them in baking as well.

This is one of my favorite breakfasts – I make it all the time and usually make enough so that I have lunch as well. Feel free to try it out yourself and experiment with your own combinations:

1 cup oats

1 cup milk

1 cup unsweetened yogurt

½ cup oat bran

½ cup unsweetened coconut flakes

½ cup fruit of your choice, chopped

Mix everything together and leave overnight. No cooking required.

Bring Back the Dairy

That's right, you can have yogurt and milk again. You should even stick to the full-fat versions. You can even add cheese back into your diet in moderation. Dairy products contain a lot of protein and can be used in place of protein in a meal. Because the protein is harder for the body to digest, the GI of these products is fairly low. There is one caveat, though – you need to look at unsweetened dairy products. That little tub of fruit yogurt can contain as much sugar as a can of soda.

Dairy can be quite useful when it comes to reducing the overall glycemic impact of a meal as a whole and can help you to feel full for longer. An added plus is that studies have shown that those who incorporate whole-fat dairy into their diet are more easily able to lose weight.

Eggs

What's not to love? Take a few minutes to prepare them and slap them on a plate for a filling and nutritious meal. Eggs are nature's original superfood. They are packed full of nutrients and healthy fats and high in protein. Boil them, fry them, bake them – just include them in your diet for a healthy boost of energy that won't skyrocket your blood sugar.

Nuts and Seeds

Okay, a few years ago I would have been laughed out of the room for suggesting that nuts should be included in order to have a healthy diet. Nuts have a bad rap because they are so nutrient dense. (I still remember running around a chair at home 40 times because I had eaten some peanuts). The good news is that nuts are really good for you and, as long as you do not eat a whole bagful at a time, they can help to regulate your sugar levels. The healthy fats contained within the nuts actually help to encourage your body to burn fat stores. The fat and protein in the nuts and seeds help make them a healthy snack for those trying to balance out their blood sugar. The caveat here is to know what portion sizes you can have – for example, a handful, or about 14 almonds, is one portion already.

You should also be sure that you get raw nuts – salted and roasted are not going to cut it here. Nuts make a great addition to that snack draw – an apple with a handful of almonds is a snack that I often make for myself.

Nut butters, as long as they are unsweetened, can make for a really good sandwich spread. (On wholegrain bread, of course.)

Red Meat

Red meat still does get a lot of bad press because of its levels of saturated fats but studies are increasingly showing that there is no causal link between saturated fats and lifestyle diseases. Where we get it wrong is that we go for portion sizes that are far too big. Your piece of meat should be no bigger than the size of your palm and no thicker than that as well. Choosing quality cuts of lamb and beef help to give you a vital dose of nutrients and the protein that you need to help maintain stable sugar levels and to repair muscle tissue.

Poultry

If red meat really is not your thing, consider adding poultry into your diet. It is high in protein and will help to slow the release of glucose into the

bloodstream. Again here the portion size is important
– be guided by the size of your palm.

Fish

You should include a serving of oily fish into your diet
at least once a week in order to ensure that your body
gets the essential fatty acids that it needs to stay
healthy. Contrary to conventional wisdom, it is not the
amount of fat in a food that makes it good or bad for
you, but rather the type of fat within that food. Fish
contains healthy fats.

Flaxseed

Flaxseed is one of the most nutritious foods on the planet. It contains healthy fats and a good deal of magnesium and is easy to incorporate into your daily diet. Simply add a teaspoon or two of crushed flaxseed to your morning cereal. (Crushing is necessary as our bodies are not able to fully digest the seeds whole.)

Olive Oil

Olive oil is one of the most stable oils when heated and is loaded with healthy, monounsaturated fats. Use it to cook with or as part of your fat allowance for the day. Fat helps to slow the absorption of glucose into the bloodstream and also helps to keep you feeling full for longer. And it can make food taste great.

Wholegrain Bread

Try and find artisanal bread at a local farmer's market. You want bread made with whole grains. Rye bread and pumpernickel are good options. Mass processed breads use a bunch of refined flours, sugars, etc. and even have taste improvers in them. Real bread should go stale in a day or two at the most.

Chia Seeds

Chia seeds are one of my firm favorites. They weren't available to me when I was growing up so I still view them as somewhat exotic. What I like about them is that they have an understated taste and can be mixed into a variety of dishes. They are a great and healthy source of protein. It is said that the ancient Aztecs would use about a tablespoon to keep them going when traveling long distances. I haven't tested that theory but I will often sprinkle them over my morning breakfast for an extra boost.

Chapter 4

Fruit and Vegetables for Diabetics

When it comes to fruit and vegetables for diabetics, you might be surprised to know that you can just about eat anything you like, as long as it is in moderation. I remember reading somewhere that a diabetic could only eat half a banana. At the time, I lived alone and so I wondered what would happen with the rest of the banana. Conventional wisdom suggests that you avoid certain fruits like bananas and grapes.

In my experience, however, as long as you are careful and pair the higher GI fruits/ veggies with protein and fats, you should be okay. For example, have the whole banana but chop it up into a tub of yogurt.

The Sweeter the Fruit

The sweeter a fruit or vegetable tastes, the higher it is in natural sugars. Whilst natural sugars are better for you than added sugars, their impact should not be negated either. Do minimize the impact by combining them with fats and proteins as detailed above.

To Peel or Not to Peel

Make it a rule of thumb to eat the peel wherever possible and you will find that you feel fuller naturally and that you are more easily able to reverse the symptoms of diabetes. The peel of the vegetable or fruit normally contains the most fiber and nutrients so if it is an option, always eat it.

Avocados

Avocados are one of my favorite foods. They have a creamy, buttery taste and can be eaten as is or mixed into guacamole. They are packed with monounsaturated fats and nutrients and can help you to lose those extra pounds that pack around the stomach.

For a diabetic, they are ideal because they have a low glycemic index and contain a lot of fiber. Half an avocado is considered one portion. If you want to keep the rest of the fruit for later, simply leave the pip in the half that is being saved and it won't turn brown.

I like to mash up an avocado with a little bit of salt and vinegar and use it on toast as a snack. Here is a recipe we use as a dip:

1/2 avocado

1 plum tomato

Juice of 1/2 lemon

1 dash salt

1/2 tsp jerk seasoning

Slice avocado into half; scoop out the flesh into a bowl and mash with a fork. Add lemon juice, salt, and jerk seasoning and combine with the same fork. Chop plum tomato and stir into guacamole.

Barley

This seems like such an old-fashioned veggie, doesn't it? Barley is a great high fiber alternative to refined rice. Keep the barley water to drink as a tonic – nothing need go to waste. Barley is packed with nutrients and will help you to feel full for longer. It has a good deal of soluble fiber to keep digestion steady.

Sweet Potatoes

This one amazed me – potatoes are not good for diabetics in general and should either be excluded or avoided. One would think that sweet potatoes, being so much sweeter, would fall under the same category. The funny thing is that they do not. They are, in fact, a good way to include some comfort food into the diet without the guilt.

They have a low glycemic index, are high in fiber and have high levels of beta-carotene in them to boot. The substances within the potatoes boost the way your body uses insulin.

Beans and Lentils

Beans and lentils are a really healthy way to get more protein and fiber in your diet and can substitute as a protein source as well. Try to buy the unprocessed beans – the tinned beans are a lot easier but tend to be packed with sodium. It is not that hard to use beans from scratch, all you need to do is to soak them at least overnight before cooking them and they make wonderful additions to soups and stews.

Here is a soup recipe that we always have on hand for cold winter nights (It serves two):

½ cup black beans (Soaked for at least 8 hours)

1 cup water

½ cup vegetable stock

One chopped onion

2 minced garlic cloves

1 teaspoon shredded ginger

1 teaspoon ground cumin

1 teaspoon ground pepper

1 teaspoon salt

Combine all the ingredients together in a slow cooker and cover with lid. Since black beans take a bit longer to cook, let this soup cook for 9-10 hours on low.

Apples and Berries

Apples and berries should be on your shopping list if you are serious about beating diabetes. Both have low levels of natural sugars and both have high levels of fiber. Eat the apples whole and unpeeled – the pectin in the apple has the effect of lowering blood sugar. The berries have a minimal impact on blood sugar – you could, for example, eat a whole bowl of strawberries without being concerned about a negative impact on blood sugar.

Chapter 5

Spice Things Up a Bit

I love a good cheeseburger and, I'll be honest, when I was looking into how to prevent myself from getting diabetes and learned that takeout would have to go, I was more reluctant to get started. What I didn't realize back then is that you can make food at home that is every bit as tasty as what you get when you order takeout and it is a good deal healthier.

Further than that, I also learned that there were some herbs and spices that could actually not only help flavor my food but that would also help to protect me against developing diabetes and to help me regulate my blood sugar levels.

Turmeric

This is actually a wonderful spice that is very popular in India. It is great for treating inflammation and the active ingredient, curcumin, has been found to be as effective an analgesic as aspirin. It is a traditional Indian remedy for treating acid indigestion and heartburn.

About a tablespoon daily is enough. Take my advice though and don't take it on an empty stomach. Mix it into your smoothie, cook with it or mix it into a half a glass of milk. This can help prevent inflammation that leads to diabetes.

Cinnamon

Plain oatmeal can take a bit of getting used to – boost the flavor by adding some cinnamon.

Cinnamon has been shown to be an effective stabilizer of blood sugar and a valuable ally in the fight against insulin resistance and Type II Diabetes. It is this effect that makes it such a valuable weight loss tool. It has been proven to be as effective in some cases as prescribed diabetes medication. Adding a teaspoon of cinnamon, a day is all that is needed to see benefits.

Cayenne Pepper

Cayenne Pepper has been proven to stimulate the metabolism, help clear away plaque in the arteries and to help reduce levels of LDL cholesterol (the one you don't want). By stimulating your metabolism, it helps you to lose more weight. In fact, all members of the chili family will help to rev up metabolism and speed up weight loss.

Ginger

Ginger is known to soothe an upset stomach but can also be instrumental when it comes to weight loss – it boosts your metabolism and can work to suppress your appetite as well. It will also help to rebalance blood glucose levels.

Cardamom

Cardamom is not really a spice that one sees used much outside of curries but this is one that can add a pleasant flavor to your food and boost the burning of fat at the same time.

Aloe Vera

Okay, so this is not a spice but I thought we could fit it in here anyway. Drinking Aloe Vera juice on a regular basis is not just good for the digestive tract, it can also help to smooth out irregular blood sugar levels and reduce inflammation and triglycerides. Some studies have found that it shows promise with the actual metabolizing of sugar as well.

Dandelion

Dandelion is never going to win any awards when it comes to flavor but it is useful in detoxing the body and helping to level out blood glucose.

Fennel

Anethole, is the "magic" ingredient in fennel helps to reduce inflammation throughout the body.

Basil

Basil, when taken after a meal, helps to reduce spikes in blood sugar. Taken on a regular basis, it will help to keep unruly blood glucose levels in check.

Rosemary

Rosemary is a good all-round tonic and promotes the digestion of fats. It also helps the body to combat inflammation.

Milk Thistle

Milk Thistle is useful when it comes to beating insulin resistance and it also helps to reduce levels of LDL cholesterol.

Garlic

This is one of Mother Nature's wonder herbs. It helps to boost immunity and reduces inflammation and plaque build-up within the body.

Stevia

This can be used safely as a natural sweetener and also as an aid in the control of blood sugar levels.

Bilberry

Full of anti-inflammatories, Bilberry also helps to improve the body's overall reaction to sugar.

Cumin

Cumin has been found to reduce blood glucose levels and help to fight cholesterol.

Sage

Sage is rich in a range of anti-oxidants and so can help prevent inflammation.

Ginseng

Taking Ginseng on a daily basis can aid in the control of blood glucose levels.

Fenugreek

This herb has a lot of fiber in it and can easily be incorporated into your daily diet if sprouted. It helps the body to process carbohydrates and can also help to slow the uptake of glucose.

Tarragon

Tarragon can help you to control hunger pangs and help to reverse insulin resistance as well.

Chapter 6

Ditch the Soda

By now you are probably aware that refined sugar is really bad for you. Did you know, however, that the average American has around 22 teaspoons of sugar a day?

Think that I am exaggerating? Open your grocery cupboard and have a look at the list of ingredients. Most tinned foods – even things like soup – will have some form of sugar in them. Not even bacon escapes – it is often cured using syrup or sugar.

Refined sugar is one of the most dangerous foodstuffs (and I use that term loosely) on the planet. It is added to most processed foods in order to improve the taste and the main problem is that it plays havoc with your blood sugar levels.

Another cause for concern is that sugar acts on the same pleasure centers in the brain that narcotics do and so you can become addicted to it just as easily.

This, combined with the impact of it on your blood sugar means that you not only get hungry faster after eating it but that you actually can become addicted to it as well.

As a result, it is far better for your health to cut it out completely.

If you must have something sweet, you can occasionally indulge in a few squares of dark chocolate – as long as you are smart about it. Stick to dark chocolate with at least 70% cocoa solids. Dark chocolate contains less added sugar than other forms of chocolate and you are consuming only a few squares a day, after a big meal so the impact on your blood sugar levels is minimal.

If having dark chocolate in the morning helps to prevent you craving sweets and feeling deprived later on in the day, the benefits far outweigh any potential risks.

The same cannot be said for sugar added to coffee, or breakfast cereals that are packed with sugar. (And believe me, a lot of the so-called healthy cereals are packed with sugar – even the bran flakes – because sugar makes them taste better.) You would be better off eating cardboard than some of the sugar-laden cereals on the market.

By avoiding too much sugar in the morning, you are reducing the chances of your blood sugar levels crashing later in the day and so are more likely to be able to stick to your healthy eating plan.

Try this experiment today, just do not add any sugar to your coffee or tea and make sure not to add it in anywhere else. Now go cold turkey for a couple of days – how did you end up feeling? Chances are good that you started out feeling as though you needed a sugar rush. Perhaps you had less energy than normal. This is a normal reaction to cutting back on your sugar intake as a whole and is basically caused by your body going into withdrawal.

If you want to cut your sugar intake completely, or want to restrict it only to the pieces of chocolate, you can choose to either go cold turkey or cut sugar out over a longer period.

The approach you choose will depend on what works best for you and how much sugar you have been consuming already.

If you have been having two sodas a day, three sugars in your coffee and sugary cereal for breakfast, it is going to be harder to kick the habit, especially if you just cut it out completely.

The cold turkey approach will work for some but not for others – the problem I have with the cold turkey approach is that you end up feeling quite horrible for about a week or so and it can be tough to keep up your motivation to stop eating added sugar.

It can also be a huge adjustment to go from having two or three spoons of sugar in your coffee to none overnight.

The good news is that you can retrain your taste-buds over time so that you gradually become accustomed to eating foods that are not as sweet.

Kicking the Sugar Habit

If you opt for reducing your sugar intake slowly, reduce it over a three-week period for optimal results. This allows you to wean yourself off sugar more slowly and helps you to avoid that nasty backlash of withdrawal symptoms.

It is important to watch out for sugar in all its forms. You would be surprised exactly how many foods do contain sugar. If a food is processed, there is a high probability that it does have added sugar. Commercial peanut butters, for example, usually have sugar in them as well.

Week 1

Halve the amount of soda that you drink and reduce the amount of sugar in your coffee/ tea by half as well. This is the week for reducing the amount of sugar you take in the form of beverages. Get rid of sugar to be used in coffee/ tea, sodas and check your creamer as well – it is likely to have sugar in it.

Week 2

Cut out the sugary snacks and desserts. If you are really battling to cope without the sugar, add in some fresh fruit snacks. One word here – whilst dried fruit is a better option than candy, it is only a slightly better option. Dried fruit does have some vitamins, minerals and fiber but also has a lot of sugar in it. The sugar in the dried fruits negates any benefits of the nutrients and fiber. You are better off eating the whole fruit – the sugars are a lot less concentrated and the water content will help you to feel full for a lot longer as well.

Week 3

Toss out processed foods and any other foods that contain high levels of added sugar. Check through your cupboards and make sure that all sugar is gone. The only sugar that you should have left in your house is in the form of natural fruits and your dark chocolate, if you are continuing with that.

The great news is that, while it may be hard to kick a sugar addiction at first, once you are over it, it becomes a lot easier to live without it. You will feel more energized, healthier and look better all for simply kicking added sugar out of your life.

You will start to see the benefits in as little as two weeks and, once you are off sugar for good, you will not really even want to go back.

Considering the negative effect that added sugar has on the metabolism, the fact that it is full of empty calories and the fact that it can actually contribute to the toxic load within the body, ditching sugar is one of the best health moves that you can make for yourself and your family as a whole.

Binge Drinking is Good

Binge drinking water, that is. You need to drink at least 8 glasses of water a day. Get yourself a water bottle and fill it up for the day ahead. Having the water ready to drink is not only a visual reminder of how much you need to drink throughout the day but it makes it a lot easier for you as well. If the water is in front of you, you are more likely to drink it. If you have to remember to go get it, you will probably forget.

If you don't like the taste of plain water, add a bit of lemon juice or some mint leaves to jazz it up a little. Always add your own flavorings. Flavored bottled water can have as much sugar in it as a can of cool drink. If you like, add a bit of plain soda water for a bit of a fizz.

It doesn't take long to get into the habit of drinking water and it so good for you.

Water should become your go-to drink. I drink about 3 liters of water a day and I love it – I cannot do without it.

It may come as a bit of a surprise to you, but you will find that your appetite starts to settle when you start out – that is because you may be mistaking hunger for thirst – making sure that you are drinking enough water every day will keep you hydrated and make it that much easier for the body to get rid of extra toxins and glucose.

Green Tea Please!

I have to be honest, I took a while to adopt the green tea fad. It wasn't that I didn't like tea, I just preferred mine with milk and green tea and milk don't work well together at all. I also felt that I had to have my morning coffee and that green tea just couldn't compete. When I tried it, I found out that I was wrong – the taste did take a bit of getting used to but the energy it gave me was great. The trick for me was to drink it cold so now I always do that – I fill a big jug with boiling water, add three teabags each of green tea and red bush tea and add a handful of mint. I let everything steep together until cool and then strain. Voila – ready to serve.

Need some more convincing?

- A lot of the bioactive compounds survive the process from tea leave to teacup. The most important of these are the antioxidants. Antioxidants help to prevent free radicals forming. Fewer free radicals mean less damage to your system. You will not appear to age as fast and will be less likely to pick up diseases.

- Cancer is still one of the biggest killers of our age. It has now been established that damage caused by oxidation is a big contributor when it comes to the growth of cancerous cells. Oxidation is caused by free radicals and these can be neutralized by antioxidants. For maximum protection, skip the milk – milk lowers the number of antioxidants present.

- Green tea has been shown to help improve the body's sensitivity to insulin and to lower the levels of sugar in the blood. A study in Japan found that you could decrease your chances of developing Adult Onset Diabetes by as much as 42%. Studies show that green tea can improve insulin sensitivity and reduce blood sugar

- Cardiovascular diseases are the biggest mass murderers the world has seen. Green tea reduces your risk of being a victim by

improving your statistics where it matters –
your LDL cholesterol, overall cholesterol and
triglyceride levels. Because of the antioxidant
abilities of green tea, LDL cholesterol is less
likely to become oxidized. This is a big one
when it comes to cardiovascular disease.
Drinking green tea regularly, without milk,
reduces your chances of cardiovascular disease
by as much as 31%.

- Catechins have anti-bacterial and anti-viral
actions as well. This is good news for your teeth
– the tea can decrease the growth rate of the
plaque-forming bacteria in the mouth. It also
helps fight bad breath.

Fruit Juices

This one may come as a bit of a surprise to you but that "healthy" fruit juice that you drink every day is anything but good for you. If you are buying a commercial brand, there is a good chance that the juice contains as much sugar in it as a soda does, and not much else in the way of nutrients. Even if you are having freshly squeezed juice, you are not in the clear – whilst you might not be adding sugar yourself, you are still getting a lot of sugar. Imagine, if it takes 4 oranges for a cup of juice, that means that you are getting the sugar from 4 oranges and little, if any, of the fiber. You may as well mainline sugar.

The only fruit juice that is acceptable to drink is freshly squeezed lemon juice. In fact, if you can manage it, it is really good for you – it helps to detoxify the body and helps to restore alkalinity. I personally cannot handle it neat so I add the juice of half a lemon to a glass of warm water first thing every morning.

Apple Cider Vinegar

Studies have shown that apple cider vinegar can help to balance blood glucose levels, encourage the body to burn fat and reduce inflammation. Drink about a tablespoonful or two in a glass of warm water about a half an hour before eating. Do this daily, twice a day for a week and then give it a break for a week.

Herbal Teas

We have already touched on some of the herbs that can be useful in the preceding chapter. If you do not want to add them to your food, an herbal tea can be a good alternative. Most herbal teas are an acquired taste so do consider sweetening them up with some Stevia or mixing two or three together until you find a combination that you enjoy.

For a standard cup of tea, you will generally use a quarter to half cup of fresh flowers/ or leaves, bruised per cup of water. Use half as much when using dried herbs.

I do just want to point out here that whilst herbal teas are natural remedies, they are not harmless and care should be taken when using them. For example, Rosemary tea could cause a miscarriage when used by a pregnant woman in the wrong doses. Always do your research first before just adopting any herbal tea regime.

Another good rule of thumb is to take the teas daily for no longer than 7-10 days and then give yourself a break of at least the same period before starting them up again. For example, Sage tea has some interesting curative properties but also has Thujone in it and this can build up to toxic levels in the body when used over a prolonged period of time.

Conclusion

Well, that about wraps it up – you should now have a much better understanding of what you should and should not do in your personal fight against diabetes. From here on out, it is up to you – you need to implement what you have learned in the book.

Most of it is just good common sense and you will know whether you are doing what is right for you or not. I generally find that if I have to start looking for rationalizations as to whether what I am doing is right or not, it probably isn't!

The bad news is that it can be a bit of an adjustment, especially when you first start out. The really great news is that it just becomes easier over time and, if you follow the advice in this book, your results will spur you on to even more success in future.

All the best for the new, healthier you!

A message from the author,

Jane Aniston

To show my appreciation for your support, Id like to offer you a couple of exclusive free gifts:

FREE BONUS!

As a free bonus, I've included a preview of one of my other best-selling books directly after this section. Enjoy!

FREE BONUS!: Preview Of

"Overcoming Anxiety - Practical Approaches You Can Use To Manage Fear & Anxiety In The Moment & Long Term"

If you enjoyed this book, I have a little bonus for you; a preview of one of my other books "Overcoming Anxiety - Practical Approaches You Can Use To Manage Fear & Anxiety In The Moment & Long Term", which goes into more detail on how you can manage anxiety safely and naturally! Enjoy!

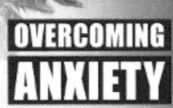

OVERCOMING
ANXIETY

PRACTICAL APPROACHES YOU CAN USE
TO MANAGE FEAR & ANXIETY IN
THE MOMENT & LONG TERM

JANE ANISTON

Short excerpt from Chapter 4

Lifestyle Changes for a Long-Term Solution

Overcoming anxiety over the long haul takes more than just a few quick fixes to quell the nerves; it requires making lifestyles changes. The changes that have to be made include getting more physically active, working on achieving optimal sleep patterns, learning to handle and minimize stress better, quitting (or at least heavily cutting down on) alcohol and smoking, cutting down on caffeinated beverages, and switching to a healthier eating habit. Long-term changes cannot happen overnight; it will require commitment and patience, as you gradually take realistic steps towards improving your mental and physical health.

Get More Active

Easily the most important and helpful thing you can incorporate into your life is a regular exercise routine. Living a sedentary lifestyle filled with stress will definitely contribute to more senseless worrying. On the other hand, frequent exercise has been proven in numerous studies to reduce anxiety symptoms. Your overall well-being will benefit due to exercise causing your body to release feel-good hormones and chemicals that will improve mood and promote relaxation.

If you have never exercised regularly in the past, you can start building the habit of being more active with simple activities that get you moving. Consider taking a 30-minute stroll around the neighborhood every morning before going to work, parking your car some distance from your destination and walking the rest of the way, taking the stairs over riding the escalator, going for a nature hike on the weekends or taking a longer than usual walk with your dog. Although these may seem like relatively minor steps, if you do them regularly you'll find yourself feeling more energized and building a higher level of self discipline. This in turn should not only allow you to move on to more strenuous exercise, but is also very likely to give you a mental boost and make you feel good about yourself.

Take Up a Formal Exercise Program

To obtain the full benefit of physical activity, consider allocating time for a formal exercise program. This involves a regular set of exercises which you have to take time out of your daily life for, such as lifting weights at the gym, attending an aerobics class, or taking up a sport. It can be challenging to commit yourself to exercising, especially when you have work-life demands to fulfill. That being said, where there is a will, there is definitely a way! Think of the money spent on health club memberships and time allocated to exercising as an investment in yourself, because your well-being matters. Again, the benefits of regular excursus have been proven by numerous studies to lead to HUGE benefits; some studies have even found that exercising regularly can be as effective as taking pharmaceutical drugs when combatting conditions such as anxiety and depression!

Try Yoga

A non-religious spiritual practice that originates from India thousands of years ago, yoga has often been touted as the comprehensive mind, body and spirit workout. These claims are far from an exaggeration though. Academic research in the western world since the 1970s has considered yoga one of the best possible treatments for depression and anxiety. Since the early 2000s, yoga has gained worldwide popularity as a fitness lifestyle practice, which has lead to it becoming a staple program offered in many gyms and health clubs. There are event studios and vacation retreats dedicated to the practice, offering courses to yogis of all levels.

In a nutshell, yoga is a system of exercise that comprises deep meditation, breathing techniques and series of physical workouts in the form of postures known as *Asana*. Some of the more orthodox yoga schools and teachers would even encourage students to incorporate the spiritual (but non-religious) elements of yoga. With consistent practice, one can reap the multiple benefits of yoga, which include:

- A calm, steady and equanimous mind

- Improved mood

- Hormonal balance

- Greater flexibility and range of motion

- Greater spinal and joint health

- Improved strength and muscle tone

- Steady weight loss and maintenance

- Lowered risk of sports injury

- Lowered risk of various chronic illnesses

- Improved self-confidence

- An overall brighter outlook on life

Those who are unfamiliar with yoga may be intimidated by the demonstration of postures that seem to require a vast amount of strength and flexibility. That should not deter you from trying out this transformative workout, because there are literally hundreds of yoga postures and they vary in difficulty. Moreover, a competent instructor – known as a guru – can guide a beginner through the practice, providing modifications to difficult postures, so the student can ease themselves into the practice.

The practice of yoga has a long history, which has branched into different traditions and styles. Certain styles are more suited to relaxation, whereas some are more physically demanding. If you intend to begin practicing yoga, take time to choose a studio and teacher that offers the style of yoga best suited to your needs.

(Chapter 4 continues in the full book)

Cognitive Behavioral Therapy

and Anxiety Disorders

Because anxiety disorders vary significantly in severity among sufferers, the treatment administered normally depends on each individual's case. One of the most common and renowned treatments for anxiety disorders is Cognitive Behavioral Therapy (CBT). It has been scientifically tested and found to be effective in hundreds of clinical trials for remedying many different mental disorders. Unlike other forms of psychotherapy, CBT is more problem-solving oriented. Patients learn specific skills that involve identifying distorted thinking patterns, modifying beliefs, relating to others differently and changing behaviors – skills which can be used for the rest of their lives.

This chapter will give you the basics on CBT, so that you will know what to expect from this treatment when seeking professional medical help for anxiety disorder.

The Theory Behind CBT

Simply put, CBT is based on the cognitive model of how the way we perceive things and situations can influence the way we feel and behave. In other words, if you interpret a situation negatively, you might feel negative emotions as a result and that in turn will lead you to behave in a certain manner. For example, someone who is obligated to attend a party might think, "This is an excellent opportunity to meet people and network!". This outlook will leave them looking forward to the event. Another person, who is less keen may think "I don't know most of the guests, so I just want to get it over and done with as quickly as possible". As you can see, it is not a situation itself that directly affects how people feel emotionally, but rather, our thoughts and perception about that situation.

When people are in distress, their perspectives and judgments are often clouded and inaccurate, causing their thoughts and imagination to run wild. CBT helps people identify thoughts that are causing them anxiety and evaluate how realistic the thoughts actually are when examined more closely. Patients then learn to change their distorted thinking patterns and adopt a more realistic approach.

(Chapter 5 continues in the full book)

Check out the rest of "Overcoming Anxiety - Practical Approaches You Can

Use To Manage Fear & Anxiety In The Moment & Long Term" on the Amazon store!

Check Out My Other Books!

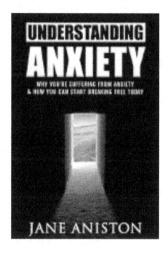

Understanding Anxiety - *Why You're Suffering From Anxiety & How You Can Start Breaking Free!*

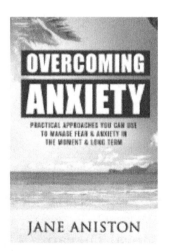

Overcoming Anxiety *-Practical Approaches You Can Use To Manage Fear & Anxiety In The Moment & Long Term*

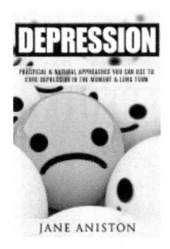

Depression - Practical & Natural Approaches You Can Use To Cure Depression In The Moment & Long Term

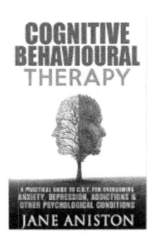

Cognitive Behavioral Therapy - A Practical Guide To C.B.T. For Overcoming Anxiety, Depression, Addictions & Other Psychological Conditions

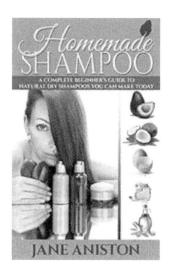

Homemade Shampoo (Includes 34 Organic Shampoo Recipes!)

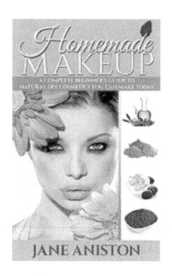

Homemade Makeup (Includes 28 Organic Makeup Recipes!)

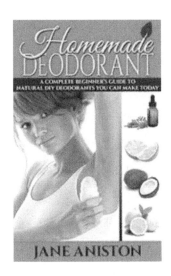

Homemade Deodorant (Includes 20 Organic Deodorant Recipes!)

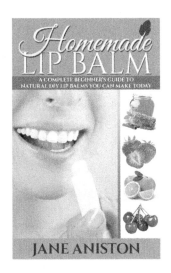

Homemade Lip Balm (Includes 22 Organic Lip Balm Recipes!)

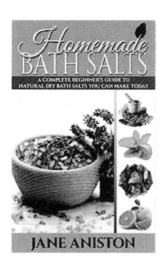

Homemade Bath Salts (Includes 35 Organic Bath Salt Recipes!)

All books available as ebooks or printed books

Made in the USA
Las Vegas, NV
26 January 2021